YOUR KNOWLEDGE HAS VALUE

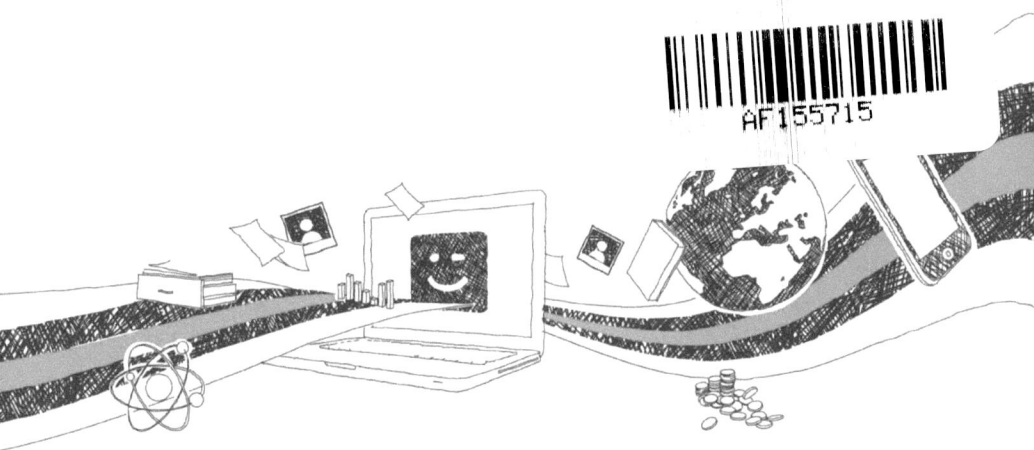

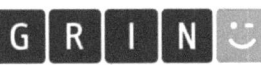

Bibliographic information published by the German National Library:

The German National Library lists this publication in the National Bibliography; detailed bibliographic data are available on the Internet at http://dnb.dnb.de .

Imprint:

Copyright © 2017 GRIN Verlag
Print and binding: Books on Demand GmbH, Norderstedt Germany
ISBN: 9783346158772

This book at GRIN:

https://www.grin.com/document/550022

James Ochieng, Slava Sobota

Exclusive breast feeding in Rusinga West Location, Kenya. Knowledge, attitude and challenges experienced by mothers with infants less than 6 months

GRIN Verlag

GRIN - Your knowledge has value

Since its foundation in 1998, GRIN has specialized in publishing academic texts by students, college teachers and other academics as e-book and printed book. The website www.grin.com is an ideal platform for presenting term papers, final papers, scientific essays, dissertations and specialist books.

Visit us on the internet:

http://www.grin.com/

http://www.facebook.com/grincom

http://www.twitter.com/grin_com

KNOWLEDGE, ATTITUDE AND CHALLENGES EXPERIENCED BY MOTHERS WITH INFANTS LESS THAN 6 MONTHS DURING EXCLUSIVE BREASTFEEDING IN RUSINGA WEST LOCATION, HOMA BAY COUNTY, KENYA.

SLAVA SOBOTA, ODHIAMBO JAMES*

Inhaltsverzeichnis

ABSTRACT

This study aimed at assessing the knowledge, attitude and identifying the challenges experienced during the practice of exclusive breastfeeding among mothers of infants less than 6 months in Rusinga West Location. This study had three specific objectives namely; to assess mother's knowledge on exclusive breast feeding, to determine mother's attitude towards exclusive breast feeding and to identify challenges faced by mother's during exclusive breast feeding practice. A descriptive cross-sectional study design was utilized. The study targeted mothers with infants less than six months of age in the location. Data was collected by administering structured questionnaires with closed and open ended questions to the targeted respondents. Data was entered into Microsoft Excel and analyzed using descriptive statistics and presented using tables and graph.

A total of 84 respondents participated and the study findings showed that majority of the respondents 98%, (n=82) had heard of exclusive breast feeding and knew what it mean. Half of the respondents, 50%, (n=42) said they had experience difficulties while breast feeding and half of the respondents 50%, (n=42) also said they have not experienced any difficulty while breast feeding. It's worth noting that majority of the respondents still face challenges such as baby refusal to breast feed, inadequate breast milk, breast tenderness, pain during breast feed and sore nipples.

Key words: Breastfeeding, exclusive breastfeeding, human Immunodeficiency Virus, maternal and Child Health, antenatal care, infant and Young Children Feeding, traditional birth attendant and community health extension worker.

1

BACKGROUND INFORMATION

According to Alade;(2013), exclusive breastfeeding is defined as infant feeding with no other food or drink, not even water, except breast milk (including milk expressed or from a wet nurse) for 6 months of life, but allows the infant to receive oral rehydration solution (ORS), drops and syrups (vitamins, minerals and medicines). The World Health Organization (2010) recommends that breastfeeding should start immediately following delivery for the baby to get Colostrum. The infant should thereafter be exclusively breastfed for up to six months of life, day and night on child's demand. During this period, no fluid including water should be given to the baby;(Ike ,2013) . Exclusive breastfeeding up to 6 months is associated with low risk of morbidity and mortality among infants (WHO, 2010). Human milk provide sufficient energy and protein to meet requirements during the first 6 months of infancy. Early introduction of foods and other liquids reduces breast milk intake, decreases the full absorption of nutrients from breast milk, and increases the risk of diarrhoea and acute respiratory infections for infants. It also limits the duration of the mother's postpartum amenorrhea and may result in shortened birth intervals;(Makena, 2014).

Despite the strong evidences available in support of EBF and extensive information on EBF for the first six months of life, its prevalence has remained low worldwide (WHO, 2010). Only about 39% of infants in the developing countries and 25% in Africa are exclusively breastfed for the first six months (Makena, 2014). The same report indicates that 6% of infants in developing countries are never breastfed (WHO, 2010). In Kenya, only 61% of children below six months are exclusively breastfed KDHS, (2014).Kenya still falls below the widely accepted "universal coverage" target for exclusive breast feeding of 90% hence there is need for more efforts and interventions to be put in place to promote EBF practice; (Odindo et al., 2014).

Globally, it is estimated that about 18% of women practice EBF while in developing countries it is 39%. The implication of this is that 39 percent of Kenyan infants are being exposed daily to an increasing risk of disease and have lowered immunity because they are given foods other than breast milk before the age of six months of age .Government of Kenya is implementing the Baby friendly hospital initiative (BFHI) that has been found to be effective in several settings in the developing world initiated through Kenya in the National Strategy on Infant and Young Child feeding; (MoPHS, 2007) .Since the introduction of BFHI there has been great improvement in the proportion of children who are exclusively breastfed from 13% in 2003,32% in 2008 and to 61% in 2014 (KDHS, 2014).However, the rates are still low hence need to find out the reasons for such. The purpose of the study is to investigate the knowledge mothers have towards exclusive breastfeeding, to identify attitudes mothers have towards exclusive breastfeeding and to identify the possible challenges experienced during exclusive breastfeeding period. The decline in exclusive breastfeeding rates despite the efforts made by the governmental and non-governmental organizations interested the researcher in identifying the reason behind these low percentiles.

PROBLEM STATEMENT.

While almost all Kenyan mothers initiate breastfeeding, 85% to 90% of them offer water and other liquids to their babies in the first month. According to KDHS, (2014) 15% of children less than 6 months are fed complementary foods, 10% consume plain water, 10% consume other milks, and 3% consume non- milk liquids during the first 6 months. Further, the same survey indicates that bottle feeding is prevalent in Kenya with 11% of children aged 6 months or younger were using a bottle with a nipple while 30% of children aged 6-9 months use a bottle with a nipple; (Jolly ,2008). This may result in increased morbidity due to unsafe preparation techniques and because a large proportion of the population do not have access to safe water sources.

JUSTIFICATION OF THE STUDY.

High infant mortality rates associated with diarrhoea, acute respiratory infections and poor responses to vaccinations that result from lack of exclusive breastfeeding can greatly be reduced if exclusive breastfeeding of infants is encouraged. This is because breast milk is the ideal nourishment for infant's survival, growth and development as it contains all the nutrients, antibodies, hormones, immune factors and anti-oxidants an infant needs to thrive; (Nekesa & Ec, 2010). In addition, the mother's antibodies in breast milk provide immunity to disease. Early supplementation is discouraged for several reasons. First, it exposes infants to pathogens and increases their risk of infection, especially disease. Second, it decreases infants' intake of breast milk and therefore suckling, which reduces breast milk production. Third, supplementary food is often nutritionally inferior to breast milk; (Makena, 2014). Exclusive breastfeeding has to be practiced in order to contribute to achieving Sustainable Development Goal number 3 which aims at ensuring healthy lives and promoting well-being for all at all stages by 2030.The findings of this research will generate information on knowledge, attitude and challenges experienced by mothers of children from less than six months during exclusive breastfeeding practice. This will from a basis for training mothers and caregivers on the importance of adhering to breastfeeding recommendations. It will also be useful to the Ministry of Health and organizations concerned with infant and young child feeding in determining the type of interventions to design in order to improve maternal and child health and promote exclusive breastfeeding among new upcoming mothers in order to realize international feeding practices of the infants .Health education on breastfeeding should also be improved in order to eliminate barriers to exclusive breastfeeding and build confidence among these mothers in order to improve on the practice.

METHODOLOGY.
Study design

This study utilized descriptive cross- sectional study design. The design was appropriate for the study as it gave an overview of the status of exclusive breastfeeding.

Study area

This study was carried out in Rusinga West Location, Rusinga Island, Homa Bay County, Kenya. Rusinga Island is situated in Mbita Sub-County along Lake Victoria. The location has 3 sub locations namely: Kamasengre East, Kamasengre West and Kaswanga sub-location. The residents of this area engage in various economic activities such as fishing, subsistence farming, livestock keeping and businesses in the local markets.

Study population and target population

The study population included all mothers currently breastfeeding and are inhabitants of Rusinga West location who are approximately while the target population included the mothers who have infants less than 6 months of age during the time of the study.

Inclusion and exclusion criteria.

The inclusion criteria was that one must a resident of Rusinga West Location, consent by signing the informed consent form attached to the questionnaire, have an infant who is 6 months old or less and be18 years and above. The study however, excluded mothers who are non-residents of Rusinga West Location, mothers who fail to consent, mothers who have babies who are above 6 months of age and mothers who are not in the age bracket of 18-45years.

Sampling technique.

Snow balling sampling technique was used in this study. This technique was suitable for this study since it was easy to carry out and included all the respondents with suitable characteristics. This technique was effective since it helped the researcher identify one suitable respondent to the next until the researcher reached his sample size in the community.

Data collection tool.

Interview administered questionnaire were used to collect the desired data. The questionnaire had both open ended questions and closed ended questions. The tool consisted of 4 components namely (demographic information, knowledge on exclusive breast feeding, attitude on exclusive breast feeding and challenges experienced on exclusive breastfeeding) which tackled the three objectives with each objective in its own component. The researcher helped the illiterate respondents in language translation. The questionnaire was administered by the researcher to the respondents. The tool was pretested 2 weeks before actual study time to ensure validity and reliability of the tool. The completed questionnaires were cleaned, coded and entered into Microsoft Excel. Descriptive statistics were used for data analysis and findings presented using graphs and tables.

RESULTS.

Distribution of respondents by age.

Majority of the respondents, 29.6% (n=25) were aged between 24-28 years, 28.2% (n=24), were aged between 29-33 years, 21.9% (n=18) were aged between 18-23 year, 10.4% (n=9) had ages between 39-43 years, 8.3% (n=7) had ages between 34-38years and 1.6% (n=1) had age between 44-49years as shown in table 4.1 below.

Table 4.1: Age of the respondents.

Age	Frequency (n)	Percentage (%)
18-23	18	21.9
24-28	25	29.6
29-33	24	28.2
34-38	7	8.3
39-43	9	10.4
44-49	1	1.6
Total	84	100.0

Age of the infants.
The ages of the infants whose mothers participated in this study is as shown in table 4.2 below. Majority of the infants aged between 3-5 months and that made a big percentage of the infants.

Table 4.2: Age of the infants.

Age of children in complete months	Frequency	Percentage Distribution
1 Month	7	8.8
2 Months	9	12.3
3 Months	16	15.6
4 Months	27	32.5
5 Months	16	20.3
6 Months	9	10.5
Total	84	100

Knowledge on exclusive breast feeding.
Almost all respondents, 98%, (n=82) had heard about exclusive breast feeding while 2%, (n=2) did not have information on exclusive breast feeding as shown in table 4.4 below.

Knowledge on exclusive breast feeding.

Response	Frequency	Percentage
YES	82	98
NO	2	2
Total	84	100

Source of information on exclusive breast feeding.

Majority of the respondents, 70%, (n=57) stated that they received the information on exclusive breast feeding from the health facilities, 25%, (n=21) received it from the media while 5%, (n=6) got the information from other sources as from community health volunteers shown in figure 4.4 below.

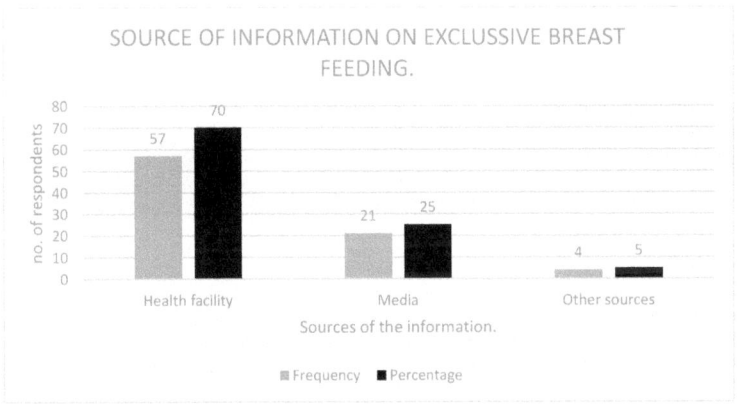

Figure 1: Source of information on exclusive breast feeding.

View on the duration of exclusive breast feeding.

Majority of the respondents 41.1%, (n=49) indicated that exclusive breast feeding should be done for six months, 15.2%, (n=18) stated four months, 11%, (n=13) stated more than six months while 3.3%, (n=4) said two months as shown in figure 4.5 below.

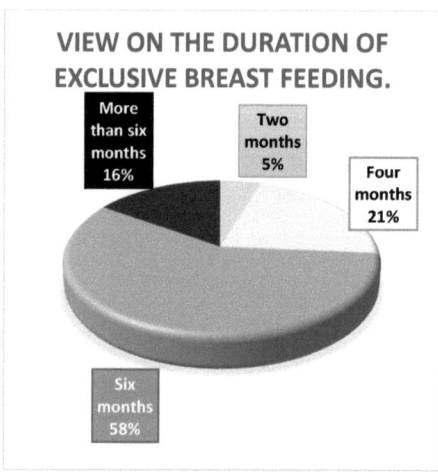

Figure 2: View on duration of exclusive breast feeding.

Position of the baby during breast feeding.
Majority of the respondents, 88% (n=74) stated that they position the baby on their lap during breast feeding while 12% (n=10) indicated that they position the baby or their arms during breast feeding as shown in figure 4.6 below.

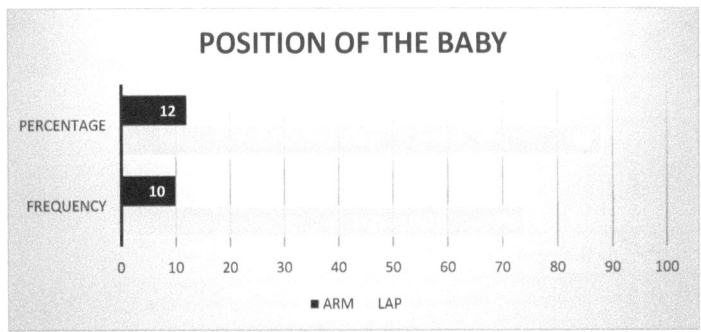

Figure 3: Position of the baby during breast feeding.

Challenges experienced during breast feeding.
Half of the respondents, 50%, (n=42) indicated that they had experienced difficulties while breast feeding while the other half of the respondents 50%, (n=42) also indicated they have not experienced any difficulty while breast feeding as shown in figure 4.6 below.

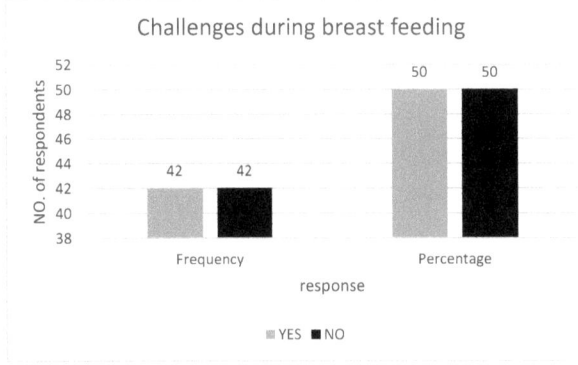

Figure 4: Challenges experienced during breast feeding.

Problems encountered during breast feeding.

Problem encountered	Frequency (n)	Percentage (%)
Inadequate breast milk	17	20.3
Baby refusing to breastfeed	3	3.5
Pain in breasts	30	35.7
Sore nipples	19	22.6
Culture does not support	1	1.1
Latching difficulty	14	16.7
Total	84	100

Alternative means when experiencing breast feeding difficulties.

Majority of the respondents, 58.3%, (n=49) indicated that they expressed and heat treated the breast milk, 19.8%, (n=17) fed the child with other foods and breast milk, 10.5%, (n=9) stopped breast feeding while 11.4%, (n=10) continued breast feeding as shown in table 4.6 below.

Alternative	Frequency	Percentage
Expressed and heat treated the breast milk	49	58.3
Continued breast feeding as usual	10	11.4

Fed the child with other food and breast milk	17	19.8
Stopped breast feeding	9	10.5
Total	84	100

DISCUSSION.

Demographic information.

Majority of the respondents, 29.6% (n=25) were young adults aged between 24-28 years. The findings also shows that majority of the respondents 51.6%, (n=43) attained primary education, 36.5%, (n=31), attained secondary education, 5.7% (n=5), and a significant number 6.3% (n=5) having attained tertiary education. This is an indicator that most of the respondents were literate. Further, 58.8%, (n=50) of the respondents are married and had a stable family. The findings further reveals that most respondents 53.8%, (n=45) were protestants an indication that they had strong religious belief in God. Moreover, majority of the participants in this study 32.5%, (n=27) had babies aged four months. This study further found out that majority of the respondents 68.8%, (n=58) lived in rural settings.

Knowledge on exclusive breast feeding.

The findings of this study shows that majority of the respondents 98%, (n=82) had heard of exclusive breast feeding and knew what it mean. This contradicts the findings of a study conducted in Nepal which found out that only 15% mothers knew meaning of exclusive breast feeding but 23.5% were practicing exclusive breast-feeding while those who did not exclusive breastfeed were 76.5%. (Shah & Raja, 2011). Moreover, a study conducted in Nigeria showed that Exclusive breastfeeding levels remain low across Africa. Between 1995 and 2010, exclusive breastfeeding in the developing world has increased from 33% to 39% (WHO, 2010).

Health facilities according to most respondents 70%, (n=57) was the chief source of information about exclusive breast feeding. This was so because they were being educated on exclusive breastfeeding whenever they visited the facilities for routine antenatal care visits. Media was the second most popular source of information about exclusive breast feeding according to the respondents. This finding is in agreement with the findings of a study conducted by Shah & Raja, 2011).

Regarding the duration that exclusive breast feeding should be carried out, majority of the respondents 41%, (n=49) indicated that it should be done for six months. However, 11%, (n=13) of the respondents indicated that it should go beyond six months. With this response, it's a clear indication that most lactating mothers in this study are aware of the minimum duration that exclusive breast feeding should be carried out. This finding however, contradicts the findings of a study conducted by WHO, (2010) in Southern Sudan which showed that most lactating mothers (65%) did not have any idea on low long exclusive breast feeding should be practiced. This variation is possibly caused by political instability accompanied by regular ethnic wars hence breast feeding mothers are not able to access health facilities where they can be enlightened on the significance of exclusive breast feeding.

Most respondents, 88%, (n=74), indicated that the baby should be on the laps while breast feeding, however, 12%, (n=10) were of contrary view. It is very true that the position of the baby during breast feeding is very important. Precise breastfeeding technique encompasses proper positioning, latching of the infant to the areola and comfort for both the infant and mother. (Shah & Raja, 2011). Several approaches of positioning tactlessly are identified, however majority of mothers embrace the single trained position. Proper positioning and latching of the nipples minimizes friction and pressure limiting sore nipples. (Koima , 2013).

All the participants in this study clearly indicated that exclusive breast feeding add a lot of nutritive value to the baby. According to Koima,(2013), Exclusive Breast Feeding (EBF) is recommended because breast milk is uncontaminated and contains all the nutrients necessary for children in the first few months of life. In addition, the mother's antibodies in breast milk provide immunity to disease, and improved cognitive development. Majority of the respondents also were of the view that exclusive breast feeding is vital in nurturing a child for a healthy growth and development.

Difficulties experienced during breast feeding.
Half of the respondents, 50%, (n=42) had experienced varying difficulty in practicing exclusive breast feeding. This case isn't different from other parts of the world since even in some developed countries, some women still finds it difficult to exclusively breast feed their infants for the

13

recommended six months. Some of the challenges experienced by the respondents while practicing exclusive breast feed include inadequate breast milk, baby refusing to breast feed, pain in breast, sore nipples, cultural barriers, breast tenderness and latching difficulty. This findings concurs with the findings of a study conducted by MacKean & Spragins,(2012), which found out that some difficulties include baby rejecting the breast, insufficient milk supply, Latching problems, nipple pain (Mastitis), pumping difficulties for instance it can be time consuming, Lack of access to effective breast pumps, finding places to pump at work/school may be difficult. Other difficulties include lack of confidence and self-efficacy, Breastfeeding is perceived as time consuming, Fatigue, exhaustion and leaking breasts. Mother's health including Smoking and other addictions, Poor diet, Hepatitis B, Post-delivery pain and recovery. Lastly infant's health that is weight loss, or failure to gain sufficient weight is also a challenge to EBF. (Makena, 2014)

Effects of the problems encountered.

Majority of the respondents, 88.0%, (n=74) said that the problems they encountered during breast feeding interfered with their breast feeding activities. In the event of difficulties in practicing exclusive breast feeding, the respondents employed other alternatives to feed their babies. Such alternatives include expressing and heat treating the breast milk in cases where the baby refuses to breast feed and feeding the child with other available light foods such as avocado.

Conclusion.

In conclusion, the exclusive breast feeding in Rusinga West Location is higher compared to the national estimates. However, it's worth noting that majority of the respondents still face challenges such as baby refusal to breast feed, inadequate breast milk, breast tenderness, pain during breast feed and sore nipples amongst others.

Recommendations.

County government of Homabay in partnership with the national government should have continual health education and promotion activities in Rusinga West Location in order to educate the breast feeding mothers of the significance of practicing exclusive breast feeding.

The health care providers in the health facilities should continuously help treat breast feeding mothers who have problems such as sore nipples by prescribing good medication for them.

REFERENCES.

Alade, O. (2013). *Exclusive breastfeeding and related antecedent factors among lactating mothers in a rural community in Southwest Nigeria.* International Journal of Nursing and Midwifery, 5(November), 132–138. http://doi.org/10.5897/IJNM2013.0111

Ike, M. . N. (2013). Utilization of Exclusive Breast Feeding Methods among Nursing Mothers in Nigeria. *Mediterranean Journal of Social Sciences,* 4(8), 69–76. http://doi.org/10.5901/mjss.2013.v4n8p69

Jolly, N. (2008). Community based peer counselors for support of exclusive breastfeeding. *Internationa lBreastfeeding Journal,* 25,101-106. Retrieved June 12, 2008, from http://www.internationalbreastfeedingjournal.com/content.

Jolly, N. and Tessa, M. (2009). *Geneva Infant Feeding Association.* Retrieved May 20, 2009, from file:///a:breast%nutrion.htm.45-67

KDHS. (2014). *Central Bureau of Statistics,*Nairobi, Kenya.

MacKean, G., & Spragins, W. (2012). *The challenges of breastfeeding in a complex world*: A critical review of the qualitative literature on women and their partners'/supporters' perceptions about breastfeeding, 65. Retrieved from http://www.albertahealthservices.ca/ps-1029951-pregnancy-2012-breastfeeding-lit-review.pdf

Makena, G. B. (2014). *factors influencing exclusive breastfeeding of children for the first six months after birth* . a case of thika level five hospital , kiambu county , kenya .56-89

N, Koima.W. J. (2013). *factors influencing adherence to exclusive breast feeding among hiv positive mothers in pumwani maternity hospital, nairobi.67-76*

Nekesa, M., & Ec, B. E. D. H. (2010). *barriers to exclusive breastfeeding and nutritional status of non – exclusively breastfed infants in eldoret municipality* , kenya, (157).

Odindo, S. J., Odindo, D. O., Alwar, J., Olayo, R., Mwayi, A., & Oyugi, H. (2014). *Demographic and Personal Characteristics Associated with Exclusive Breastfeeding among Lactating*

Mother in Siaya County of Nyanza Province in Kenya, 2(4), 45–49. http://doi.org/10.13189/ujfns.2014.020401

Shah, T., & Raja, S. (2011). ¡ *Original Article Knowledge and practice of mothers regarding breast feeding* : a hospital based study. Health Reniania, 9(3), 194–200.

WHO (2010) *Infant and young child feeding.* (n.d.).

YOUR KNOWLEDGE HAS VALUE

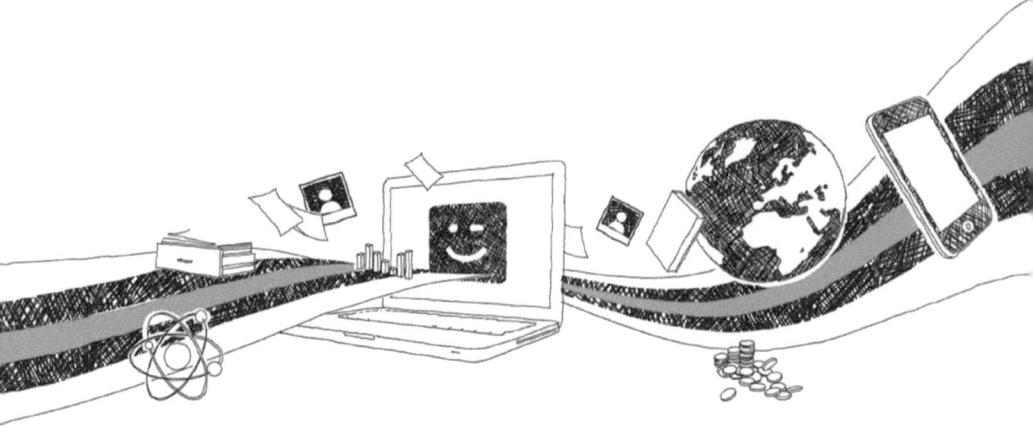

- We will publish your bachelor's and master's thesis, essays and papers

- Your own eBook and book - sold worldwide in all relevant shops

- Earn money with each sale

Upload your text at www.GRIN.com and publish for free

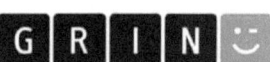